Low-Water High-Energy Weight Loss

Ching H. Wu, PhD
Li. Ac.; Diploma OM; MS OM; Dipl Ac NCCAOM; PhD Chem Eng

A revolutionary dietary concept

Healthy diet and lifestyle

Effective weight loss plan

August 05, 2012
February 8, 2016
December 20, 2018

Low-Water High-Energy Weight Loss
Author: Ching H. Wu

ISBN-13:
       978-0615841731 (Ching H. Wu)

ISBN-10:
       0615841732

Library of Congress Control Number: 2013915582

Acknowledgments

To all my patients for giving me the privilege to treat them in the last 18 years. And through these years of patient care, I was able to study and assess the etiology of obesity and refine the Low-Water High-Energy Weight Loss Plan.

To YungHuo Zhung, a self-taught Chinese herbalist who was well known as "the one who can cure a cold overnight". His practice was a crystallization of his experience using the teaching of Zhang ZhungJins's Shan Han Lung. His advice to curtail consumption of fresh fruits, raw vegetables and cold drinks has had a profound influence on my own practice in Chinese Medicine and on the development of this weight loss method.

To my wife, Tihn, for adopting the low-water high-energy diet plan for our family. As a result, members of our family have not experienced weight problems.

In the early 1990's Tihn had fibromyalgia. She was severely depressed by the constant and decimating pain and by realizing there is no effective cure in sight. At that time, I was a petroleum engineering professor at Texas A&M University and was illiterate in health issues. Nevertheless, I promised Tihn that with my scientific and engineering knowhow I could find some ways to alleviate her pain and decided to enroll in the Texas Institute of Oriental Medicine & Acupuncture. With help from instructors and fellow students, I treated Tihn's ailment with acupuncture and Chinese herbs. Tihn felt better and stronger week after week and in two years her fibromyalgia was effectively cured. A year later, I became a licensed acupuncturist in the State of Texas.

To Dr. Ruth Yang, who is a medical doctor from Shanghai, China, and is very well versed in acupuncture. She was able to relieve Tihn's pain temporarily with each acupuncture treatment. Her encouragement to pursue my goal of developing a human engineering skill is much appreciated.

To my daughter, June, for her support and assistance in completing this book.

To my daughter, Chemi, and twin grandkids, Preston and Kiki, for their love and willingness to follow components of the Low-Water High-Energy Plan.

To George Young and many patients who inspired and encouraged me to write this book.

To the numerous authors of articles posted on the world wide web. The information provided from their individual or aggregate research was very helpful in building a case for the Low-Water High-Energy Diet.

To Crystal Long for organizing the interior of the book into a good format.

To Teresa Matteson for her skillful editing on portions of the book.

Contents

Tables

Formulas

1. Introduction

In spite of enormous efforts to fight obesity, millions of Americans are overweight and getting fatter. Countless diet plans, public school programs, billions of dollars spent on research and medical expenses have not helped the obesity epidemic.

Obesity is a disease of excess accumulation of water and fat. The excess water and fat accumulation can cause numerous other diseases including high blood pressure, diabetes, systemic pain, kidney failure, heart disease, limited mobility, and depression. Annually, billions of dollars are spent on treating these obesity related diseases.

In a recent conversation, my good friend George Young raised the subject of obesity in American society. He asked me why, as an engineering professor and acupuncturist, I would discourage "at least eight glasses of water a day" for those who want to lose weight. I told him that water is the major factor in weight gain. George pointed out that water does not have calories, so why would it be a big factor in the weight problem. I explained that a calorie has no weight, but a mass, like water, does. Excess water accumulation is the major cause of obesity. Then, he asked if I applied that principle to help my patients lose weight. I admitted that I have done so for the past 15 years. Many of my patients lose three to five pounds in the first week of my diet plan. After a few weeks of steady weight loss and noticeable pain reduction, they are feeling better.

I suggest that the solution to excess water and fat accumulation is a mass (weight) balance problem. The customary diet routine of calorie counting may or may not be effective for weight loss unless it incorporates weight balance. A weight balance is prerequisite to an effective weight loss plan. So, forget counting calories alone if you plan to lose weight. Instead, work on weight balance and count pounds and ounces.

We will succeed in eliminating obesity if we have the will to control our body weight balance - how much mass (food and water) we allow to come into our body and how much mass (stool, urine, perspiration, and respiration) we have to discharge from our body every day.

2. Weight Gain Mechanisms

Many of my patients admit that they gain weight easily. They have jokingly told me that they can gain weight just by drinking water. I always looked them in the eye and told them "It is not a joke to me. Water alone can make you fat!" (See Appendix A, page 42)

From a scientific standpoint, what else would make my patients gain tens and hundreds of pounds? These patients always indicated to me that water should not make them fat, calories do. As a practitioner of human engineering, I told them I disagreed about calories making them fat. Water has mass that can put weight on you. A calorie (heat energy) is weightless and cannot be the culprit. In Chinese Medicine the excess water and fat (tan yin) accumulation is the main cause of obesity. In Chinese, "tan" means phlegm; "yin" means drink; both are non-functional body fluids.

In order to help my patients lose weight, I started to analyze the weight gain mechanisms. I consider the human body to be an open thermodynamic system surrounded by the universe. As asserted by the basic medical philosophy of Chinese Medicine, the heaven and human are one. The human body's function and health are intimately affected by its environment: food, drink, atmosphere (air, humidity, pressure, and pollutants), wind, cold, heat, dwellings (shelter, commode, shower, and air conditioning), other humans, organisms, etc. The basic chemical and physical sciences tell us that in a system consisting of a human body and its surroundings, mass is conserved, momentum is conserved, and energy is conserved in spite of complicated human metabolism, chemical reactions, and physical and emotional activities. It is obvious that the weight gain is caused by the excess accumulation of mass (water and non-aqueous food substance) when there is an excess mass intake or insufficient mass discharge, or both. Remember that the heat energy (calories) has little to do with weight gain except empowering human activities.

Let us analyze weight gain by the principle of water mass conservation. Within a specific time period, the mass of water (in beverages and in food) taken into the human body plus the mass of water generated from bio-fuel (lipids, carbohydrate, and protein) oxidation, minus the mass of water leaving the body equals the accumulation of water mass inside the body. This is a very simple concept that can easily be put into practice. If we measure the amount of water taken in, the amount of water generated from oxidation of bio-fuels (Appendix A), and the amount of water excreted, we will determine how much water our body has gained or lost. Similarly, a mass conservation can be made for the non-aqueous portion of food substance. If we identify the factor that causes weight gain, we can eliminate the factor and subsequently lose weight.

To further illustrate the water conservation concept, we can use the bath tub as a model. A bath tub is like a human body with a mouth (faucet) and lower orifice (drain). The faucet, just like the human mouth, puts water into the system. During the filling period, the drain is closed and the faucet turned on. Like a human body consuming liquid, the filling tub gains water (mass or weight). Since there are no calories (carbohydrate, protein, fat) in water this weight gain is completely independent of caloric intake. While the faucet is on, if the drain leaks comparable to the human urine and stool and there is vaporization from the water surface comparable to human respiration and perspiration, then the water related weight gain will ease. If the faucet is turned off and the drain left open with moderate vaporization, the water level in the tub will decrease for an overall loss in water (weight). The tub gains or loses weight regardless of the water temperature or calorie content.

The human body is much more complicated than a bath tub. Nevertheless, the mass conservation principle applies. The water mass coming in, plus the water mass generated within the human body (product of bio-fuel consumption), minus water mass discharged (urine, respiration from the lungs, and perspiration from skin) must equal water weight gain or loss.

In addition to water retention from liquid intake, the non-aqueous food (such as non-aqueous carbohydrates, proteins, fats, and other organic compounds and minerals) retention can also contribute to the weight gain. The non-aqueous food retention is equal to the non-aqueous food intake minus the sum of non-aqueous food in stool, the non-aqueous food converted to body mass as human cells, and the non-aqueous food consumed as bio-fuels. Since the non-aqueous food substance is about 25% of total food and drink intake, the contribution of non-aqueous food to weight gain is relatively small.

How much water does the bath tub contain after the first fifteen minutes? It is not easy to figure out the right answer. The same question can be asked for the human body. And obviously, it will be harder to get the right answer since in addition to what we eat and drink, the calculation must factor in losses from urine, stool, respiration and perspiration, and the water produced from bio-fuel consumption. The right answer for the human body equation holds the key to effective weight management. To help you determine the right answer for your body, I provided a model for these calculations (Appendices A, B, and C) and developed the Low-Water High-Energy Diet Plan (Appendix D).

3. **Water Factor**

The human body is about 65 to 70% water; similar to the water weight percent of earth. Therefore, water is the dominant component in our body weight. If we want to lose weight, we need to focus on managing the water.

Many of my patients who want to lose weight told me that their doctors or nutritionists advised them to drink at least eight glasses of water a day. I asked my patients "Did they tell you why you need to drink at least eight glasses of water a day?" The answer was "to flush out bodily wastes and toxins" or "you are dehydrated". I suggested that body wastes and toxins cannot be flushed out by urination alone. And I mentioned that with the excess water you already have in your body, it is unlikely you will be dehydrated any time soon. I asked them if they lost weight drinking at least eight glasses of water a day. The answer was always "No, I feel lousy and I am gaining weight!"

Excess water accumulation indicates that the kidney's excreting capacity has been exceeded. Too much water intake is damaging to the kidneys and the kidney function that could result in frequent urination and urinary incontinence. According to Chinese Medicine, the excess water can dilute the blood and body fluids and retard the blood and body fluid circulation causing local or systemic pain, edema, and obesity. As the overloaded kidneys become dysfunctional, they can subsequently affect the function of other vital organs such as Heart, Lung, Liver, Spleen, etc., causing a multitude of illnesses.

As previously mentioned, water is not always ingested in liquid form. Foods like vegetables and fruits have water contents that range from 75 to 95%. From that perspective, eating those vegetables and fruits is like drinking water. Various meats contain at least 50% water. The amount of water in foods consumed in our daily diet can account for up to 25% of our total daily water intake.

One of our family friends is an intelligent and well-educated woman. During a dinner party, she mentioned that she was gaining weight. I asked how much liquid she drank in a day. Her reply was that she hardly drank anything: two cups of coffee and a soft drink per day. She said that she watched her diet carefully: a small bowl of cereal with milk for breakfast, an apple for lunch, and a reasonable dinner. I noticed after an eight-course dinner, she had several servings of gelatin. I asked if she knew that the gelatins are more than 80% water. She said she was aware of that. I told her that she was really drinking the gelatin rather than eating it. She insisted that she was eating the gelatin. The point is that she may have more water intake in a day than she thought.

Through years of acupuncture practice, I have observed a common symptom with obese patients and patients with leg and foot edema. After acupuncture, water oozed out of the needled area in their legs. This implies that the excess water in my patients' legs is in an extracellular free water state. The excess water is being stored between the soft tissues. The free-state water between the tissues can be removed from the body more easily than the water that is inside the cells of fat, muscles, bones, etc. Can you imagine what would happen to the obese patients if they drink 8 or more glasses of water a day? This recommendation for water intake is ill-informed and it promotes and perpetuates obesity epidemic.

Water exists as a solution or micellar solution in the human body. It is present both in lean body tissues and fat body tissues as intracellular and extracellular water. The water content of these tissues may be inferred from the water content in animal tissues: in lean tissues of pork, chicken, beef, and fish ranging from 65 to 72% and in fat tissues from 15 to 40%. As inferred, human fatty tissues may contain a large amount of water. So, when we say we lose fats as we slim down, 15 to 40% of the "fat" lost may be water.

It is easier to lose water weight than to break down fat (lipids) and other tissues such as muscle, tendons, and bones. The loss of water weight early in a diet program will provide encouragement to the dieter to gradually lose fatty tissues.

Water is a big factor in weight control. It is important to understand the mechanisms of water retention in order to lose weight effectively. The following is recommended for body water control:

1. Limit water intake to a minimum; drink water only when you feel thirsty or dehydrated.
2. Keep your digestive tract, pulmonary system, and body as warm as possible. Drink warm and hot drinks, ingest warm and hot meals, inhale warm air, avoid cold air directly from air conditioning, take a hot shower every day, and warm your hands and feet when they are cold or when you feel they are cold.
3. Dress warmly all the time; when sleeping, keep your neck, forehead, and head warm with small towels.
4. Have at least one bowel movement a day.
5. Have regular urinations.
6. Exercise regularly to increase respiration and perspiration.

4. The Myth of Calorie Balance

From the perspective of an engineering professor and scientist, I believe it is a myth that in order to lose weight, you simply need to consume fewer calories than your body utilizes. It is also a myth when people say that being overweight is a result of an energy imbalance – eating too many calories and doing too little exercise. Such claims have no basis in basic sciences. I have sympathy for my patients who have been misled by such myths for so long.

The basic sciences tell us that a calorie (little) is a unit of energy. It is equivalent to the amount of heat needed to increase the temperature of one gram of water at one atmospheric pressure from 4 degrees Celsius to 5 degrees Celsius. It represents the amount of energy that has the potential to do work. The basic sciences also tell us that the energy is released (exothermic) or absorbed (endothermic) when atomic bonds are broken or altered in chemical reactions or physical processes. The totality of energies is conserved in the chemical reaction or physical process, but, the heat energy (calorie) may not.

Food calories (combustion energy, a food calorie is 1,000 multiple of a little calorie) are determined with the assumption that the carbon and hydrogen in food are fully oxidized in a calorimeter. The heat released from the exothermic reactions is measured as the energy content of the food. It is a good indicator of food nutrition value. But, as the heat energy released is weightless, it has little to do with weight gain. Further, in the human body environment, the food's carbon and hydrogen are unlikely to be fully oxidized. There are always excess calories from food, more than our body would normally use. This heat energy (calorie) imbalance has little to do with weight gain.

High calorie foods do not automatically put weight on people. The excess calories are simply not released and are not automatically converted to fats. The combustion (oxidation) of carbohydrates (sugars), proteins, and lipids (fats) in foods releases a lot of calories. The balance between the calories in food consumed and the calories used in human body functions and activities has no relevance to weight control. Excess calories (heat energy) may be stored as internal energy. Therefore, oversupply of calories may not necessarily lead to weight gain, but oversupply of mass like water, does contribute to weight gain. Simply put, according to the calorie count, intake of <u>one gram</u> of sugar will give you <u>four food calories</u>. However, the intake of <u>a glass</u> of water will give you <u>zero food calories</u>, but will give you <u>two hundred and twenty seven grams</u> of weight. For weight control, I would rather take one gram of sugar than take a glass of water. I definitely do not want to take more than 8 glasses of water a day (4 pounds water; 0 food calories.)

Instead of dwelling on the caloric content of foods as in the customary approach, Chinese Medicine recognizes that every herb or food has the potential to be exothermic, neutral or endothermic. The level of such potential is indicated by a non-quantitative scale of "hot", "warm", "neutral", "cool", and "cold". Proper use of the herbs or foods with these characteristics can be a great help for weight control.

The human body does need energy conversion to provide potential energy (heat) for adequate metabolism, physical activities, respiration, and perspiration. Respiration and perspiration promoted by energy conversion are crucial mechanisms for discharging body fluids and waste.

While a calorie balance does not indicate weight gain or loss, a mass (weight) balance of food and water does – as in the accumulation of water in the bathtub. Therefore, a mass (weight) balance approach, not a calorie balance is the key to a successful weight control program.

5. Low-Water High-Energy Diet

The Low-Water High-Energy Diet was developed based on the weight gain mechanisms and the water mass balance principle. In this diet, oral intake must have the lowest water content possible and yet provide enough energy to release waste products and body fluids. Within a given time period, the total mass (pounds) of food and drink intake must not exceed the sum mass (pounds) of discharges (urine and stool) and expended body fluids (moisture from skin and lungs, sweat, saliva, nasal mucous, and tears). If you diligently follow the Low-Water High-Energy Diet Plan, you will not gain weight for the rest of your life.

First, I will discuss the low-water part of the diet. Often, you hear the suggestion that if you want to lose weight, you should take in plenty of high-water content foods such as fruits, vegetables, soups, etc. You have also heard that you need to drink at least eight glasses of water per day. This means you turn on the faucet at a high rate and the tub is filling up quick. These suggestions are contrary to the water mass conservation principle to lose weight. Therefore, they are not helpful for weight loss. Instead, based on the mass conservation principle, you should take in low-water content foods such as bread, rice, meat, dried fruits, canned fruits, and cooked vegetables. You should also curtail beverages such as water, juice, coffee, tea, soft drinks, and beer as much as possible.

Table 1 shows the water content of fresh and cooked vegetables. The water content of fresh vegetables ranges from 74 to 96% by weight. A large portion of our daily water intake can come from fresh vegetables. The water content data for the cooked foods was obtained using a crucible, a porcelain coated stainless steel wire gauze, an electronic weight scale, and a gas burner. When cooked, the vegetable contracts and releases part of its water. The water weight percentage of the cooked vegetables is 10 to 15% less than uncooked vegetables. Cooked or preserved (canned) vegetables are preferred over fresh raw vegetables.

Table 1. Water Content of Fresh and Cooked Vegetables

Vegetables	Weight % Water	
	Fresh*	Cooked **
Lettuce	96	77
Cucumber	96	92
Celery	95	81
Zucchini	95	78
Tomato	94	94
Cabbage	93	82
Spinach	92	83
Cauliflower	92	83
Broccoli	91	78
Carrots	87	72
Onion	82**	81
Potato	79	72
Peas	79	64
Corn	74**	60

*Cooperative Extension Service, University of Kentucky

**Wu crucible analysis data

Table 2 shows the water content of some cooked foods and dairy products. Bread has low water content, therefore is highly recommended for the Low-Water High-Energy Diet. Rice and meats having moderate water content are good choices as well. French fries have low water content (36%) but may have high oil content. If the total amount of French fries consumed in a meal is relatively small, they may also be a good choice. Bean curd, milk, yogurt, and gelatin have high water content, therefore, only a minimal amount is recommended.

Table 2. Water Content of Cooked Foods

Cooked Foods	Weight % Water**
Bread	37
Steamed rice	63
Stirred fried beef	54
Lamb	64
Salmon	67
Kelp trout	74
Fried chicken	70
Fried egg	67
Bacon	27
Steak fat	18
Hamburger	54
French fries	36
Potato salad	68

Cooked Foods	Weight % Water**
Bean Curd	80
1% fat milk	87
Vanilla ice cream	60
Oatmeal cookies	6
Crackers	7
Peanut butter	6
Yogurt	82
Gelatins	85

**Wu crucible analysis data

Table 3 shows the water content of fresh and dried fruits. The water content of fresh fruits ranges from 74 to 92%. A minimal amount of fresh fruits is recommended in the Low-Water High-Energy Diet. Instead, canned, cooked or processed fruits are preferred. Dried fruits have much lower water content (only 25 to 30% by weight). They are highly recommended to substitute for fresh fruits. Fruit juices have a high-water content (>90%), and therefore, are not favored in the Low-Water High-Energy Diet.

Table 3. Water Content of Fresh and Dried Fruits

Fruits	Weight % Water

	Fresh*	Dried**
Watermelon	92	--
Strawberries	92	15
Grapefruit	91	17
Cantaloupe	90	12
Peach	88	30
Cranberries	87	18
Orange	87	25
Pineapple	87	12
Raspberries	87	6
Apricot	86	10
Blueberries	85	15
Plum	85	32
Pear	84	30
Apple	84	22
Grapes	81	19
Cherries	81	15
Banana	74	6

*Cooperative Extension Service, University of Kentucky
**Estimates from food label (Wu)

Many patients have gained weight by consuming a large quantity of fresh fruit every day. For example, there is the watermelon diet. Since the water content of watermelon is more than 90% by weight (see Table 3), it is equivalent to drinking a large amount of sweetened water. Instead of eating watermelon, people are actually "drinking" it. Many of these patients have puffy round faces, bulging limbs and hips, and protruding pot bellies. After I advised them to reduce watermelon consumption, they experienced immediate weight loss. One of my female patients loved to eat watermelon. She had watermelon for breakfast, lunch, and dinner. She kept gaining weight and did not know what to do. She felt sluggish and tired all day. I asked her to follow the Low-Water High-Energy Diet and stop eating watermelon. She lost three pounds in a week and felt better.

The second part of the diet involves high energy, warm or hot food and drink. In Traditional Chinese Medicine, food that has high energy potential tends to increase the rate of metabolization, heat generation, respiration, and perspiration. It helps the release of body fluids like sweat and mucous. Table 4 lists the non-quantitative energy potential of foods.

Table 4 Energy Potential of Foods

Vegetable	Energy potential
Squash	Warm
Garlic	Warm
Green onion	Warm
Coriander	Warm
Yam	Neutral
Carrot	Neutral
Lettuce	Cool

Vegetable	Energy potential
Cauliflower	Cool
Broccoli	Cool
Tomato	Cool
Winter melon	Cool
Celery	Cool
Spinach	Cool
Mushroom	Cool
Sea weed	Cold
Bitter melon	Cold
Bamboo shoot	Cold
Lotus root	Cold

Fruit	Energy potential
Peach	Warm
Hawthorn	Warm
Grape	Neutral
Pear	Cool
Orange	Cold
Water melon	Cold
Apple	Cold

Fruit	Energy potential
Banana	Cold

Cereal	Energy potential
Sorghum	Warm
Rice	Neutral
Soy bean	Neutral
Sesame	Neutral
Wheat	Cool
Buck Wheat	Cool
Mung bean	Cool

Protein	Energy potential
Beef	Warm
Lamb	Warm
Duck	Warm
Pork	Neutral
Chicken	Neutral
Goose	Neutral
Quail	Neutral
Egg	Neutral

Protein	Energy potential
Tofu (bean curd)	Cold

Sea Food	Energy potential
Eel	Warm
Sea cucumber	Warm
Salmon	Neutral
Bass	Neutral
Steel head	Neutral
Carp	Neutral
Sun fish	Neutral
Turtle	Neutral
Frog	Cool
Crab	Cold
Oyster	Cold
Clam	Cold

Nuts	Energy potential
Walnut	Warm
Chestnut	Warm
Pine nut	Warm

Nuts	Energy potential
Almond	Neutral
Peanut	Neutral
Sunflower seed	Neutral
Filbert	Neutral

Condiment	Energy potential
Pepper	Hot
Ginger root	Hot
Cinnamon	Hot
Vinegar	Warm
Peanut oil	Neutral
Honey	Neutral
Sugar	Neutral
Salt	Cold
Soy sauce	Cold

Beverages	Energy potential
Wine (alcohol)	Warm
Milk	Neutral
Water	Neutral

Beverages	Energy potential
Tea	Cool
Fruit juice	Cold

High energy potential (warm or hot natured) foods and drinks are preferred in the Low-Water High-Energy Diet. Low energy potential (cool or cold-natured) foods must be cooked or heated prior to consumption. The cooking and heating of cold natured foods raises their energy potential especially when hot natured condiments like ginger root, pepper, and cinnamon are added.

Cold drinks and foods with a temperature much lower than human body temperature are discouraged from the Low-Water High-Energy Diet. Avoid cold beverages and cold foods as much as possible, especially straight out of the refrigerator. Cold natured food/drink and cold temperature food/drink interfere with the body's ability to release excess fluid.

The processed (canned) and dried fruits not only have lower water content, they have a relatively higher metabolic potential ("warm" as compared to the "cold" nature of fresh fruits). These "warmer" foods are much better than fresh fruits for promoting physical and emotional activities leading to a greater release of body fluid.

A woman with pain in her back, knees, and shoulders came to see me recently. She was five feet four and weighed 250 pounds. I told her that her pain most likely was from being overweight - too much water that dilutes the blood and slows the circulation. I advised her to be on the Low-Water High-Energy Diet and gave her herbs that promote circulation. In a week, she lost four pounds and was almost pain free. She went on to lose 14 pounds in 4 weeks and had more energy.

The Low-Water High-Energy Diet is a no cost and no pain diet. You do not have to pay extra money for diet pills or prepackaged meals. You can eat and drink practically anything you want. The only stipulation is to choose food and beverages that are low in water content and high in energy potential. Food and drinks that are laden with water or have low energy potential (cold) will hamper your ability to lose weight.

6. **Proper Exercises**

Proper exercises are very important in weight management. Activities involving the mind and body promote burning of bio-fuels. These activities increase body metabolism, respiration, and perspiration which help expel bodily wastes and fluids. Increased expenditure of bio-fuels, respiration, and perspiration can certainly contribute to weight reduction.

Consistent respiration and perspiration are not only crucial for the release of body fluid for weight control, they are also important for the release of body heat for temperature control. If the mechanism of skin perspiration is hampered by atmospheric cold temperatures, the stagnated body fluids and body wastes could affect the lung respiration and poison body tissues. In addition to weight gain, this could also lead to catching a cold or flu, asthmatic cough, and wheezing. Proper exercises promote respiration and perspiration; thereby help to relieve these symptoms. Some Chinese herbal medicines restore the stagnated skin perspiration for the treatment of cold, flu, asthma, and weight gain.

Proper exercises can be physical exercise, mental exercise or emotional exercise as long as they can increase respiration and perspiration. Proper exercises do not necessarily have to be strenuous activity. The individual has a variety of choices. It can be as simple as walking up and down the stairs. It can be planting and pruning in the flower garden. Tai Chi Chuan and yoga are also excellent examples. Simple diaphragm breathing (Chi Gong) which induces muscle contraction and extension is an effective form of exercise. Intense reading of mental and emotional content may also qualify. The important point is that the exercise should be enough to promote quick respiration and light sweating. After exercises, you need to drink the proper amount of water to replenish your body fluids.

For many years, I have intently studied the game of tennis and it has been my major form of exercise. Often, I played tennis in my sleep. I also practice Tai Chi Chuan and routinely do shadow Tai Chi Chuan in bed before I go to sleep. I do diaphragm breathing (Chi Gong) on a regular basis, even when I am teaching classes or playing tennis. These mental, emotional, and physical exercises help me to perspire effectively. By following the principles of the Low-Water High-Energy Diet and proper exercises, I have not gained more than five pounds in the last 50 years.

Normal respiration through the mouth and nose may discharge 0.58 to 1.59 pounds of body fluids per day (Appendix B). It may increase substantially for people who do strenuous exercises like athletes. Perspiration through the skin may discharge 0.75 to 1.50 pounds of body fluids a day. For those who do a lot of manual exercises, it could increase at least four folds. If proper exercises can help you respire and perspire 5 pounds of body fluids a day, an equivalent to 10 glasses of water, you may effectively lose weight or control your weight gain. How much water you have respired and perspired can be determined by the weight balance system described in Appendix C.

Normal consumption of bio-fuels a day can be estimated from the amount of carbon dioxide respired (Appendix A and Appendix B). If we can estimate additional carbon dioxide respired a day due to exercises, we can estimate the additional bio-fuels consumed due to performing the proper exercises.

Proper exercises increase the body's interaction with the environment. They help improve motor skills, agility, and awareness of environments. They help maintain healthy physical, mental, and emotional balance.

Proper exercises help to reduce the body fat and body fluid. Drinking after exercises does not interfere with weight control; it replenishes water loss from respiration and perspiration.

7. **Helpful Herbs**

Chinese herbs are useful for weight loss in many ways. They are excellent thirst-quenchers, laxatives to help with constipation, diuretics to increase urination, and diaphoretics for respiration and perspiration. Herbs are very helpful for supplementing a weight loss program using the Low-Water High-Energy Diet.

When formulated properly by a knowledgeable Chinese herbalist, the herbs should be effective with minimal to no side effects. Also available are off-the-counter Chinese herbal supplements for public use. Do not take these herbs without consultation with a licensed practitioner of Chinese Medicine.

Major symptom: Thirst

Often there are people who want to lose weight and complain about extreme thirstiness resulting in the need to drink a lot of water. If they continuously consume a large amount of water, they have little chance of losing weight. Many herb formulas can help quench thirst and reduce the desire for water. The cause of thirstiness can be determined from differential disease pattern analysis using associated symptoms. The following herbs are available for a variety of disease patterns that cause dry mouth and thirstiness.

Thirst-quenchers:
Liu Wei Di Huang Wan (Six Ingredient Rehmannia Pill)

Dry mouth; difficult urination; night sweat; difficult sleep; cold sweat; low-grade fever.

Zhi Bai Di Huang Wan (Anemarrhena-Phellodendron-Rehmannia Pill)

Dry mouth; difficult urination; night sweat; difficult sleep; cold sweat; low-grade fever; **red face**.

Wu Ling San (Five Ling Powder)

Dry mouth; difficult urination; lassitude; sluggishness; nausea; edema.

Zhu Ling San (Polyporus Powder)

Dry mouth; difficult urination; anxiety; sleeplessness; cough; bloody urine.

Suan Zao Ren Tang (Sour Jujube Decoction)

Dry mouth; difficult urination; anxiety; difficult sleep; night sweat; palpitation; light headedness.

Major symptom: Constipation

One or two bowel movements a day is normal for the average healthy person. If you have one bowel movement every two days, you are constipated and this will lead to difficulty with weight control. People with one bowel movement every three or four days definitely need help. The following herbs are useful laxatives for different disease patterns.

Laxatives:

Tiao Wei Chen Qi Tang (Smooth stomach and Qi Decoction)

Constipation; stomach pain; sore throat; cold sore; bad breath.

Ma Zi Ren Wan (Hemp Seed Pill)

Constipaton; dry stool; frequent urination.

Tong Bian Wan (Pass stool pill)

Constipaton; dry stool; abdominal distention.

Major symptom: Difficult urination

Diuretic herbs help to promote the release of fluid through urination. Some of the thirst-quenchers can also be used as diuretics.

Diuretics:
Liu Wei Di Huang Wan (Six Ingredient Rehmannia Pill)

Difficult urination; night sweat; difficult sleep; cold sweat; low-grade fever; dry mouth.

Zhi Bai Di Huang Wan (Anemarrhena-Phellodendron-Rehmannia Pill)

Difficult urination; night sweat; difficult sleep; cold sweat; low-grade fever; red face; dry mouth.

Wu Ling San (Five Ling Powder)

Difficult urination; lassitude; sluggishness; nausea; edema; dry mouth.

Zhu Ling San (Polyporus Powder)

Difficult urination; cough; blood in urine; anxiety; sleeplessness; dry mouth.

Major symptom: Low perspiration

The following herbs are diaphoretics that promote perspiration. The herbs are used when the patient has difficulty releasing sweat.

Diaphoretics:
Ren Shen Bai Du San (Ginseng Expelling Poison Powder)

No sweating; cough; stiff neck; stuffy nose; congested chest.

Xin Su San (Prunus-Perilla Leaf Powder)

No sweating; chill; cough; stuffy nose; clear phlegm.

Shen Su Yin (Ginseng-Perilla Leaf Decoction)

No sweating; chill; fever; stiff neck; headache; sticky phlegm.

Chinese herbs are less effective for people who drink water, fluids, and alcohol excessively. If you follow the Low-Water High-Energy Diet Plan, the herbs can greatly help your weight loss efforts.

8. Weight Balance

Weight balance is very important in implementing the Low-Water High-Energy Weight Loss Plan. Measurement for weight balance requires fairly accurate scales. It is worthwhile to invest in two scales: one for measuring body weight (accuracy to 0.05 pound, about $180, designated as "A scale") and one for measuring food (accuracy to 0.01 ounce (0.1 gram), about $60, designated as "B scale"). Another option may be to borrow or rent these scales for about 3 days when you start the weight loss plan. Or, you can just follow the dietary plan using a regular bathroom scale (accuracy to 0.1 pound, about $40, designated as "C scale").

Weigh yourself every day at the same time each day. Over a 24 hour period of time, you want to figure out if there has been a gain or loss of weight. The simplest method is to subtract the weight at the end of 24 hours (W_e*, Appendix C, page 50) by the weight at the beginning (W_b*). The difference (W_c) between the two weights tells you how much weight you lost or gained in a day. The sign convention here is, <u>negative value indicating weight loss</u>; <u>positive value indicating weight gain</u>. Keep a daily record of your measurements so you can monitor your progress on the weight loss program.

For those of you interested in exercising your math skills, I have included some formulas for calculating the weight balance (Appendix C). Many quantitative items used in the formulas can be measured using A scale. For example, taking a weight before breakfast and a weight after the breakfast, the difference is the weight of your breakfast. Similarly, you can determine the weight of lunch, dinner, urination, defecation, respiration and perspiration when resting, respiration and perspiration when sleeping, and respiration and perspiration when exercising. If the amount of water respiration and perspiration (W_{rpw}) is low, then proper exercises would be recommended. If water perspiration (W_{pp}) is low and the person is constipated, then laxatives and diaphoretics may be prescribed to increase daily discharges (stools and perspirations).

We can complete a total water weight balance to determine the change in water weight (accumulation, W_{cw}) in a 24-hour period. This change in water weight represents the contribution of water to weight gain or weight loss per day and shows the need for a water management program.

Similarly, a non-aqueous food weight balance can determine the contribution of the non-aqueous portion of your intake to weight gain or loss.

The Low-Water High-Energy Diet was developed on the assumption that water retention (accumulation) is the dominant factor for weight gain or weight loss. Since the human body is 65 to 70% water and the total food intake is about 70 to 75% water, this assumption would appear to be valid.

9. Positive Reinforcements

A positive attitude is necessary for starting a weight loss plan. You must be mentally prepared and willing to change your eating habits. Any initial weight loss will reinforce more positive thinking about weight control.

It is also important to have a continuous interest in eating and drinking better. Being more choosy and selecting better tasting food and drink should make the healthy diet more attractive. Dining with family and friends who can help your weight management will make the diet more enjoyable. Realizing a healthy diet will encourage you to continue following the weight loss plan.

It is also very important to continue a routine exercise and refine the exercise to be more enjoyable and more satisfying. An athletic club or a local gym would be a good place where you could find a variety of exercises and a host of people enjoying the same activities. In one of these athletic clubs, I have found participation in groups for tennis, line dance, and Tai Chi to be very enjoyable.

Some people may feel that practicing with a tennis ball machine is boring and unproductive. On the contrary, I think it is the most challenging and gratifying device I have ever used to improve my tennis shots, concentration, agility, and health. In addition to challenging myself to make every shot better than the previous one, I also try to incorporate my knowledge in Tai Chi martial arts for improving my game. In less than five minutes with the ball machine, I start to sweat and in less than an hour, I get plenty of exercise with a healthy loss of body fluids. I have regularly practiced tennis with a ball machine for the last three years and it is an important part of my weight management.

I believe that most of you who follow this weight loss plan will find that:

1. You feel lighter.
2. You breathe better.
3. You sleep better.
4. You have more mobility.
5. You have less joint, muscle, and back pain.
6. You can easily put on clothes.
7. You can easily tie shoe laces.
8. You can live a more enjoyable lifestyle.
9. You feel healthier; have less cold, flu, allergy, etc.

10. You feel happier.

10. Healthy Diet and Lifestyle

The following is the Low-Water High-Energy Weight Loss Plan suggested for every patient in my clinic. These guidelines are good for all patients, not just for those who would like to lose weight. An example Low-Water High-Energy Diet Plan is shown in Appendix D (page 62).

Drinks

- **Prefer warm (at least room temperature) or hot drinks.**
- **Drink only when you feel thirsty or dehydrated. Excessive drinking is discouraged.**
- **Cold drinks or iced products are discouraged. A small amount of cold drink for enjoyment is okay.**
- **A small amount of alcohol is fine.**

Foods

- **Prefer foods that are low in water content and "warm" natured.**
- **"Cold" natured foods should be cooked and heated up.**
- **Eat only up to 70 to 80% of fullness.**
- **Take in a small amount of snacks if needed.**
- **Fresh vegetables and raw meats are discouraged. A small amount of fresh vegetables for enjoyment is acceptable.**
- **Prefer "warm" natured, dried, and canned fruits.**
- **Fresh fruits are discouraged. Small amounts of fresh fruits for enjoyment are fine.**

Enjoyable Meals

- Make sure you have a healthy digestive system. Seek medical help if you have: a poor appetite or an uncontrollable appetite, thirstiness, dry mouth, chapped red lips, canker sores, constipation or diarrhea.
- Choose food and beverage that you like and enjoy your meals.
- Eat and drink with family and friends.

Weight Records

- Weigh yourself at a specific time of the day.
- Keep a written daily record of your weight.
- Use your record to adjust your intake and select proper exercises.
- Challenge yourself to find ways to lose and maintain weight.

Proper Exercises

- Find an interesting and challenging exercise or exercises that you enjoy.
- Set aside time every day to do the exercise(s) till you feel a light sweat.
- Challenge yourself to do better or excel in the exercise(s).
- Do exercises with family and friends.

11. Time Frame

A weight loss program should be carried out over a long period of time, six months to a year or more. Weight control and maintenance is done over a life time, not just for one to two weeks. Anyone who is interested in starting a dietary program should have a long term goal. One should determine how much weight to lose and how soon. The time table for losing weight should be realistic, achievable, and comfortable.

Many of my patients lost four to five pounds in the first week after taking up the Low-Water High-Energy Diet Plan. However, my recommendation would be to lose weight more slowly. It is generally accepted that a one to two pound weight loss per week is safe and longer lasting. I encourage you to stay on my diet plan long term even after you reach your goal weight. The Low-Water High-Energy Diet is not only effective for losing weight, but also for maintaining your weight and good health.

I am fortunate to have a wife who followed the Low-Water High-Energy Diet Plan for over fifty years in our household. We are in our 70's now and still in good health. Our weight has not deviated more than five pounds since our earlier years. It is my hope that everyone who follows this diet plan will also enjoy good health. Life is too brief to suffer with excess weight, pain, and limitations. This dietary program will help you change your lifestyle. I wish for all of you a fully active and optimal life.

12. Other Applications

Cold drinks and foods with a temperature much lower than human body temperature are not recommended on the Low-Water High-Energy Diet. Food and drink that is cold in temperature cools off the esophagus, stomach, and small intestines. The lowered temperature, even a few degrees, slows down the metabolism and causes accumulation of water in the surrounding areas. In severe cases, the colder temperature can suppress the perspiration of the entire body (chills.) Adjacent to the mouth and esophagus are the nose, sinuses, throat, and part of the lungs. Water accumulation in these areas can cause sinus congestion, excess phlegm, stuffy chest, and asthma. I believe cold drinks and foods are one of the major causes of increasing asthma in the United States, especially in children because they are more susceptible. Around the stomach and small intestines, excess water accumulation can cause upset stomach, indigestion, and weight gain. It is my belief that cold drinks and foods are one of the major causes of obesity in the United States, especially in younger people.

The Low-Water High-Energy Diet is not only good for weight loss, it is also helpful for people with respiration and perspiration related problems. For example, one of my patients was a ten year old boy who had chronic and severe asthma since birth. The boy had a stuffy nose, phlegm, chest congestion, and eczema. He was also slightly obese. He loved cold drinks and was allowed to drink as much as he wanted. Routinely before bed time, he had a glass of cold orange juice. His asthma was so severe he needed to visit the emergency room regularly. I put him on the Low-Water High-Energy Diet and gave him herbs that would help him perspire through his skin and lungs. A week later, he breathed better, slept better, and cleared his eczema. A few months later, I was told that the boy had not been back to the ER ever since.

The Low-Water High-Energy Diet is also helpful for people having joint/muscle pains caused by excess fluids (weight) obstructing the channels (circulation). One female patient could not walk into my office without help. She had severe pain in her left hand, both shoulders, both thighs, and left foot. She could not sit down on my office chair because of the pain. Her blood pressure was 195/103 and pulse rate 107. She was slightly obese. Her diet included cold drinks, fresh salads, fresh fruits, and ice cream. I put her on the Low-Water High-Energy Diet and gave her herbs for stress and high blood pressure. I also treated her with acupuncture and advised her to see her family doctor for hypertension. Three days later she slept better with less pains. Her blood pressures went down to 170/96 with a lower heart rate of 95. Ten days later, she had a lot less pain and was able to use her fingers again. Her blood pressure and pulse rate continued to decrease with dietary changes, herbs, and antihypertensive drugs. Four weeks later she had lost four pounds and her blood pressure dropped to 144/80 with a pulse rate of 80. She was now practically painless.

Recently, I used the water weight balance principle to help one of my patients from a life threatening scenario. The patient was admitted to a hospital for colon surgery. The surgery was successful, but the anesthetic and morphine paralyzed her intestines and urinary tract. She had unbearable abdominal pain from bloating. The only treatment for the pain was to prescribe more morphine. The nurse told my patient the pain may be caused by intestinal accumulation of gas. I was suspicious that the gas alone could not cause the severe bloating and asked the nurse to weigh the patient. Her weight was 115 pounds. The initial weight on admission was 105 pounds. My patient gained 10 pounds in just a few days! Since admission to the hospital, she was given a lot of intravenous fluid, but did not have much urination and no bowel movements. I knew right away that the abdominal bloating was partially caused by the accumulation of water. A bladder scanner indicated that a liter of fluid had accumulated in the patient's bladder! When the nurse applied a catheter, the container overflowed with urine. The patient experienced rapid pain relief after her bladder was drained. I believe this is not an isolated case. My suggestion is that in addition to routinely taking the vital signs of surgery patients, their weight should also be monitored. A water weight balance can be used to adjust the IV rate of fluids to avoid excessive water accumulation.

Other applications for the Low-Water High-Energy Diet are far reaching and extend beyond the weight loss plan. Special consideration should be given to the water content in food and drink. I believe this is important enough to suggest that all food and beverage labels should include the water weight percent. This information can help people make the right choices for regulating their weight and maintaining their health.

Appendix A. Estimate of Bio-fuels Consumed

The majority of non-aqueous food intake is lipid, carbohydrate, and protein. These are the source of energy for human physical, mental, and emotional activities and substances for cell and tissue replacement. These substances providing energy are called bio-fuels.

How much bio-fuel is consumed and how much non-aqueous food is stored as fat each day becomes an important issue in weight control.

While daily food and drink consumed varies from person to person, we can assume an initial estimate of 6.6 pounds per day per average adult: 1.4 pounds breakfast, 1.8 pounds lunch, 2.1 pounds dinner, and 1.3 pounds snacks. A good estimate of the non-aqueous portion of the 6.6 pounds is 26%, i.e. 1.7 pounds. The water portion will be 4.9 pounds which includes 2.6 pounds from drinks and 2.3 pounds from foods.

 Biofuels are mainly composed of carbon, hydrogen, and oxygen. If fully oxidized, one gram of biofuel would generate an average of about 5 food calories. If an average adult needs 2,200 food calories per person per day, 0.97 pounds bio-fuels would be consumed. The required 0.97 pounds bio-fuels are far less than the 1.7 pounds of non-aqueous food intake of the average adult per day. This explains the inadequacy of calorie balance on weight control. If we must cut down the daily intake to 0.97 pounds from 1.7 pounds, it would be unbearable.

Fortunately, not all the non-aqueous foods consumed are necessarily converted to calories each day. Part of the non-aqueous foods is used to replace cells and tissues and part is discharged as stools. If we assume the non-aqueous portion of daily stools discharged weighs 0.39 pounds, we have 0.34 pounds of non-aqueous foods for cell and tissue replacement and for storing in our body.

The 0.97 pounds biofuels require 1.06 pounds of oxygen to completely oxidize to produce 0.58 pounds of water and 1.45 pounds of carbon dioxide. Most of the carbon dioxide produced must be respired through the mouth and nose and that can be estimated from the amount of air breathed through the lungs (Appendix B, next page). The 0.58 pounds of water from the bio-fuel consumption must be factored into the water weight balance. This means that the average adult needs to get rid of at least 5.5 pounds of water per day (2.6 pounds from drinks, 2.3 pounds from foods, and 0.58 pounds from bio-fuel consumption) to achieve zero water gain. If the average adult drinks at least 8 glasses of water (4 pounds) a day, his body needs to work very hard to get rid of the additional 1.4 pounds of water (4 pounds minus 2.6 pounds). This may explain why many obese patients complain that they can gain weight by drinking water alone!

Since calorie balance as popularly used for weight control disregards water weight balance, it is inadequate for providing a guideline for weight loss. The important issue is how the average adult can get rid of the 6.6 pounds of daily intake for a perfect weight balance.

Appendix B. Estimate of Water and Carbon Dioxide Respired

How much water moisture respired through the lungs per day may be estimated from the air inhaled and exhaled per day.

The moisture content of inhaled air is lower than that of the air exhaled. Relative humidity and atmospheric temperature dictate the moisture content of the air inhaled. The moisture content of the exhaled air depends on the body temperature and is usually fully saturated with water.

We can estimate the water moisture respired each day with the following assumptions:

Atmospheric temperature	50 °F, 70 °F, 90 °F
Relative humidity (%)	30, 40, 60, 80,100
Body temperature	98 °F
Inhaled air composition (on dry air basis)	
Nitrogen	78.970 volume %
Oxygen	21.000 volume %
Carbon dioxide	0.030 volume %
Exhaled air composition (on dry air basis)	
Nitrogen	77.800 volume %
Oxygen	18.000 volume %
Carbon dioxide	4.200 volume %

Tables 5, 6, and 7 show the water moisture respired each day in pounds per day per person. Variables that influence the amount of water moisture exhaled include the breath capacity (volume of air in cubic centimeters), rate of respiration, atmospheric temperature, and relative humidity.

Table 5. Water Moisture Respired (lbs/day), Temperature 50 °F

300 cc per breath

Rel humidity, %	12 breath/min	16 breath/min	20 breath/min
30	0.474	0.632	0.790
40	0.466	0.621	0.776
60	0.448	0.598	0.747
80	0.431	0.575	0.718
100	0.414	0.551	0.689

400 cc per breath

Rel humidity, %	12 breath/min	16 breath/min	20 breath/min
30	0.632	0.843	1.054
40	0.621	0.828	1.035
60	0.598	0.797	0.996
80	0.575	0.766	0.958
100	0.557	0.735	0.919

500 cc per breath

Rel humidity, %	12 breath/min	16 breath/min	20 breath/min
30	0.790	1.054	1.317
40	0.776	1.035	1.293
60	0.747	0.996	1.245
80	0.718	0.958	1.197
100	0.689	0.919	1.149

600 cc per breath

Rel humidity, %	12 breath/min	16 breath/min	20 breath/min
30	0.948	1.264	1.580
40	0.931	1.241	1.552
60	0.896	1.195	1.494
80	0.862	1.149	1.436
100	0.827	1.103	1.278

Table 6. Water Moisture Respired (lbs/day), Temperature 70 °F

300 cc per breath

Rel humidity, %	12 breath/min	16 breath/min	20 breath/min
30	0.446	0.595	0.743
40	0.428	0.571	0.713
60	0.392	0.522	0.653
80	0.355	0.473	0.592
100	0.318	0.424	0.531

400 cc per breath

Rel humidity, %	12 breath/min	16 breath/min	20 breath/min
30	0.595	0.793	0.991
40	0.571	0.761	0.951
60	0.522	0.696	0.870
80	0.473	0.631	0.789
100	0.424	0.566	0.707

500 cc per breath

Rel humidity, %	12 breath/min	16 breath/min	20 breath/min
30	0.743	0.991	1.239
40	0.713	0.951	1.189
60	0.632	0.870	1.088
80	0.592	0.789	0.986

| 100 | 0.531 | 0.702 | 0.884 |

600 cc per breath

Rel humidity, %	12 breath/min	16 breath/min	20 breath/min
30	0.892	1.189	1.487
40	0.856	1.141	1.427
60	0.783	1.044	1.305
80	0.710	0.947	1.184
100	0.639	0.849	1.061

Table 7. Water Moisture Respired (lbs/day), Temperature 90 °F

300 cc per breath

Rel humidity, %	12 breath/min	16 breath/min	20 breath/min
30	0.393	0.524	0.655
40	0.357	0.476	0.595
60	0.284	0.379	0.474
80	0.211	0.281	0.351
100	0.136	0.182	0.227

400 cc per breath

Rel humidity, %	12 breath/min	16 breath/min	20 breath/min
30	0.524	0.699	0.874
40	0.476	0.635	0.794
60	0.379	0.506	0.632
80	0.281	0.375	0.468
100	0.182	0.242	0.303

500 cc per breath

Rel humidity, %	12 breath/min	16 breath/min	20 breath/min
30	0.655	0.874	1.092
40	0.595	0.794	0.992
60	0.474	0.632	0.790

80	0.331	0.468	0.586
100	0.227	0.303	0.378

600 cc per breath

Rel humidity, %	12 breath/min	16 breath/min	20 breath/min
30	0.786	1.049	1.311
40	0.715	0.953	1.191
60	0.569	0.759	0.848
80	0.422	0.562	0.704
100	0.273	0.364	0.456

For the assumed conditions, the amount of water respired per day per person ranges from 0.136 to 1.580 pounds. The amount of water respired is higher when the atmospheric temperature and relative humidity are lower. When exercising, the rate of breathing increases substantially, thereby, more water will be respired. We can use the tables to estimate the amount of water respired each day. For example, when the atmospheric temperature is 70 °F, relative humidity is 60 per cent, air volume is 500 cc per breath, and rate of breathing is 12 breaths per minute at rest, the estimated amount of water respired is 0.632 pounds per day. If the rate of breathing is increased to 20 due to proper exercises, the amount of water respired is increased to 1.088 pounds per day.

Table 8 shows the amount of carbon dioxide respired each day per person.

Table 8. Carbon Dioxide Respired (lbs/day)

cc per breath	12 breath/min	16 breath/min	20 breath/min
300	0.768	1.024	1.279
400	1.024	1.365	1.706
500	1.280	1.706	2.133
600	1.536	2.048	2.560

The carbon dioxide respired is a function of the amount of air respired (cc per breath and breath/min) in a day. It is not affected by the atmospheric temperature and the relative humidity. The carbon dioxide respired ranges from 0.768 pounds per day to 2.560 pounds per day.

Appendix C. Weight Balances

Symbols

* Weight that can be measured or estimated.

Gross Weight Balance

W_b*	weight of body at the beginning of 24-hour period
W_e*	weight of body at the end of 24-hour period
W_c	change in weight over a 24-hour period (negative value indicating weight loss)
W_f*	weight of food (solid or semi-solid) intake during the 24-hour period
W_d*	weight of drink intake during the 24-hour period (assuming drink is 100% water)
W_i	weight of total intake during the 24-hour period
W_{dis}	weight of total discharge during the 24-hour period (stool, urine, perspiration, respiration, secretion)
W_u*	weight of urine during the 24-hour period (weighing before and after urination)
W_s*	weight of stool during the 24-hour period (weighing before and after defecation)
W_{rpt}	weight of respiration and perspiration (water vapor, sweat, carbon dioxide, nitro oxide, and salts) during the 24-hour period

Water Weight Balance

W_f*	weight of food (solid and semi-solid) intake during the 24-hour period
W_{fs}*	weight of the non-aqueous parts in food intake during the 24-hour period
W_{fw}*	weight of the water in food intake during the 24-hour period
W_s*	weight of stool during the 24-hour period
W_{ss}*	weight of solid in stool during the 24-hour period
W_{sw}*	weight of water in stool during the 24-hour period
W_{pCO2}*	weight of carbon dioxide respired during the 24-hour period
W_{rpw}	weight of respiration and perspiration of water vapor (including sweat) during the 24-hour period
W_{pr}*	weight of water vapor respired during the 24-hour period
W_{pp}	weight of water vapor perspired during the 24-hour period
W_{fo}*	weight of water from the bio-fuel oxidation
W_{cw}	change in water weight (water gain or water loss) during the 24-hour period

Non-aqueous Food Weight Balance

W_{cs}	change in non-aqueous parts during the 24-hour period

13. Gross Weight Balance

The body weight balance for a 24-hour period is:

Formula 1. Body Weight Balance

$$W_e^* - W_b^* = W_c$$

W_b^*	body weight at the beginning of 24-hour period
W_e^*	body weight at the end of 24-hour period
W_c	change (accumulation) in weight over a 24-hour period (negative value is a loss and positive is a gain)

Formula 1 is the easiest to follow for checking weight gain or loss in a day. All you need to do is measure W_b^* and W_e^*. Maintaining a record for W_b^*, W_e^* and W_c is important for charting your progress and should be done daily.

If you are really serious about weight control, you need to use Formulae (2), (3), and (4) to determine the weight of respiration and perspiration (W_{rpt}). The total intake is specified by Formula 2.

Formula 2. Total Intake

$$W_i = W_f^* + W_d^*$$

W_i	total intake during the 24-hour period
W_f^*	food intake during the 24-hour period
W_d^*	weight of drink intake during the 24-hour period (assuming drink is 100% water).

Formula 3 is the calculation for the weight of total discharge, W_{dis}.

Formula 3. Total Discharge

$$W_{dis} = W_i - W_c$$

W_{dis}	total discharge during the 24-hour period
W_c	weight gain or loss obtained from Formula 1

All discharges are negative values.

Then, use Formula 4 to calculate the weight of daily respiration and perspiration, W_{rpt}.

Formula 4. Daily Respiration and Perspiration

$$W_{rpt} = W_{dis} - W_u{}^* - W_s{}^*$$

W_{rpt}	weight of respiration and perspiration (water vapor, carbon dioxide, nitro-oxide, sweat, and salts) during the 24-hour period
$W_u{}^*$	weight of urine during the 24-hour period
$W_s{}^*$	weight of stool during the 24-hour period

Perspiration is an important factor suggesting the need for proper exercise. For example, if someone does not perspire much, proper exercise should be done to promote perspiration. If a person perspires a lot every day, a prescription for curtailing $W_f{}^*$ (food) and $W_d{}^*$ (drink) and promoting $W_u{}^*$ (urine) and $W_s{}^*$ (stool) should be in order.

14. Water Weight Balance

In addition to total weight balance, we need to make water weight balance to determine the gain or loss of water. The daily food intake is defined in Formula 5.

Formula 5. Daily Food Intake

$$W_f^* = W_{fs}^* + W_{fw}^*$$

W_f^*	food intake during the 24-hour period
W_{fs}^*	non-aqueous parts in food intake during the 24-hour period
W_{fw}^*	water in food intake during the 24-hour period

Formula 6 is the calculation for the weight of daily stool, W_s^*.

Formula 6. Daily Stool

$$W_s^* = W_{ss}^* + W_{sw}^*$$

W_s^*	weight of stool during the 24-hour period
W_{ss}^*	weight of solid in stool during the 24-hour period
W_{sw}^*	weight of water in stool during the 24-hour period

In practice, we can estimate W_{fw}^* as 70-75% of W_f^* (70% meat and 75% veg) and W_{sw}^* as 65-90% of W_s^* (firm 65%, soft 70%, loose 80%, and 90% watery.)

The amount of water respired and perspired in a day can be calculated from Formula 7.

Formula 7. Daily Water Respiration and Perspiration

$$W_{rpw} = W_{rpt} - W_{pCO2}* \times 0.273$$

W_{rpw}	weight of water respired and perspired (including sweat) during the 24-hour period
$W_{pCO2}*$	weight of carbon dioxide respired during the 24-hour period (estimated from Appendix B)

Here, 0.273 is the carbon to carbon dioxide weight ratio.

The amount of water perspired in a day can be calculated from Formula 8.

Formula 8. Daily Water Perspiration

$$W_{pp} = W_{rpw} - W_{pr}*$$

W_{rpw}	weight of water respired and perspired (including sweat) during the 24-hour period
$W_{pr}*$	weight of water respired during the 24-hour period (estimated from Appendix B)
W_{pw}	weight of water perspired during the 24-hour period

Formula 9. Change in Water Weight (Accumulation)

$$W_{cw} = (W_{fw}* + W_{d}*) - (W_{sw}* + W_{u}* + W_{rpw}) + W_{fo}*$$

$W_{fo}*$	weight of water from bio-fuel oxidation
W_{cw}	change in water weight (water gain or water loss) during the 24-hour period

We can complete a total water weight balance to determine the change in water weight (accumulation) in a 24-hour period. This change in water weight represents the contribution of water to weight gain or weight loss per day and shows what needs to be adjusted in water management.

15. Non-aqueous Food Weight Balance

Formula 10 shows the change in solid (non-aqueous) weight that represents the contribution of solids to weight gain.

Formula 10. Contribution of Non-aqueous Food to Weight Gain

$$W_{cs} = W_c - W_{cw}$$

W_{cs}	change in non-aqueous parts during the 24-hour period

W_c, W_{cw}, and W_{cs} are very important data for producing an effective weight loss program.

The Low-Water High-Energy Diet was developed on the assumption that W_{cw}, change in water weight, is a dominant factor for weight gain or weight loss.

16. Example Weight Balances

Two major estimates were necessary to complete the example weight balance. One is the amount of water respired from the lungs, 0.785 pounds per day, as calculated from Appendix B assuming 400 cc per breath, 12 breaths per minute, and 60 percent humidity at 73 °F of atmospheric temperature. The other estimate was 1.024 pounds per day of carbon dioxide respired under the above assumed conditions that generated 0.41 pounds of water produced per day from consuming 0.69 pounds of bio-fuels (Appendix B).

Table 9. Example Weight Balances

Factor	Description	Lbs
$W_b{}^*$	weight of body at the beginning	139.08
$W_e{}^*$	weight of body at the end	138.99
W_c	change in weight ($W_e{}^*$ - $W_b{}^*$) (- = weight loss, + = weight gain)	-0.09
$W_f{}^*$	weight of food intake	2.68
$W_d{}^*$	weight of drink intake (assuming drink is 100% water)	3.20
W_i	weight of total intake during the 24-hour period ($W_f{}^*$ + $W_d{}^*$)	5.88
W_{dis}	weight of total discharge (stool, urine, perspiration, respiration) (W_i – W_c)	5.97
$W_u{}^*$	weight of urine (weighing before and after urination)	3.60
$W_s{}^*$	weight of stool (weighing before and after defecation)	0.74
W_{rpt}	weight of respiration and perspiration (water vapor, carbon dioxide, sweat, etc.) (W_{dis} - $W_u{}^*$ - $W_s{}^*$)	1.63

Table 10. Example Water Weight Balance

Factor	Description	Lbs
W_f^*	weight of (solid and semi-solid) food intake	2.68
W_{fs}^*	weight of non-aqueous parts in food intake	1.07
W_{fw}^*	weight of water in food intake ($W_f^* - W_{fs}^*$)	1.61
W_s^*	weight of stool	0.74
W_{ss}^*	weight of solid in stool	0.17
W_{sw}^*	weight of water in stool ($W_s^* - W_{ss}^*$)	0.57
W_{pCO2}^*	weight of carbon dioxide respired (Appendix B)	1.02
W_{rpw}	weight of respiration and perspiration of water vapor (including sweat) ($W_{rpt} - W_{pCO2}^* \times 0.273$)	1.35
W_{pr}^*	weight of water vapor respired (Appendix B)	0.79
W_{pp}	weight of water vapor perspired (including sweat)	0.56
W_{fo}^*	weight of water from bio-fuel oxidation	0.41
W_{cw}	change in water weight (water gain or water loss) (Formula 9)	-0.30

Table 11. Example Non-aqueous Food Weight Balance

Factor	Description	Lbs
W_{cs}	weight change in non-aqueous part $(W_c - W_{cw})$	0.21

Results showed that the amount of water respired and perspired (W_{rpw}) was 1.35 pounds, and the amount of water perspired from the skin (W_{pp}) were 0.56 pounds. For the day, the subject person lost 0.30 pounds of water (W_{cw}, a negative value) while gaining 0.21 pounds non-aqueous foods (W_{cs}, a positive value) resulting in a net loss of 0.09 pounds (W_c, a negative value).

17. Blank Weight Balance Sheets

The following blank weight balance sheets are for you to record your daily weight balance.

Factor	Description	Lbs
$W_b{}^*$	weight of body at the beginning	
$W_e{}^*$	weight of body at the end	
W_c	change in weight ($W_e{}^* - W_b{}^*$) (negative value indicating weight loss)	
$W_f{}^*$	weight of food intake	
$W_d{}^*$	weight of drink intake (Assuming drink is 100% water).	
W_i	weight of total intake during the 24-hour period ($W_f{}^* + W_d{}^*$)	
W_{dis}	weight of total discharge (Stool, urine, perspiration, respiration) ($W_i - W_c$)	
$W_u{}^*$	weight of urine (weighing before and after urination)	
$W_s{}^*$	weight of stool (weighing before and after defecation)	
W_{rpt}	weight of respiration and perspiration of water (water vapor, sweat, etc.) ($W_{dis} - W_u{}^* - W_s{}^*$)	

Factor	Description	Lbs
W_f*	weight of (solid and semi-solid) food intake	
W_{fs}*	weight of the non-aqueous parts in food intake	
W_{fw}*	weight of the water in food intake (W_f* - W_{fs}*)	
W_s*	weight of stool	
W_{ss}*	weight of solid in stool	
W_{sw}*	weight of water in stool (W_s* - W_{ss}*)	
W_{pCO2}*	weight of carbon dioxide respired (Appendix B)	
W_{rpw}	weight of respiration and perspiration of water vapor (including sweat) (W_{rpt} - W_{pCO2}*x 0.273)	
W_{pr}*	the weight of water vapor respired (Appendix B)	
W_{pp}	the weight of water vapor perspired (including sweat)	
W_{fo}*	the weight of water from bio-fuel oxidation	
W_{cw}	change in water weight (water gain or water loss)	
W_{cs}	weight change in non-aqueous part (W_c − W_{cw})	

Appendix D. Example Low-Water High-Energy Diet Plan

Most American meals are 75 to 85 per cent water by weight. The water content of snacks is close to 90 per cent. The water content of these meals needs to be curtailed to less than 75 per cent. Cold drinks should be minimized or avoided altogether.

The following meal plans are recommended for the Low-Water High-Energy Diet.

Table 12. Breakfast

Group	Food	Wt (oz)	H_2O factor	H_2O wt (oz)
Grain	Bread	4.00	0.37	1.48
	Or cereal, rice			
Meat	Lean meat	4.00	0.54	2.16
	Boiled or fried egg	2.00	0.67	1.34
Vegetable	Stir-fried lettuce	4.00	0.75	3.00
	(or steamed lettuce)			
Fruit	Canned	3.00	0.80	2.40
	(or preserved)			
Drinks	Hot tea	6.00	1.00	6.00
	(or water, coffee)			
Total	oz	23.00		16.38
	lbs	1.44		1.02
Water content				71%

It is the individual's choice of food for each category in the breakfast. In place of bread, one may choose cereals, pancakes, waffles, muffins, oatmeal or rice. Milk, syrup, jam, jelly, honey, butter may be added.

In the lean meat category, one may choose grilled or baked chicken, pork, beef, turkey or fish. Eggs may be boiled, fried or scrambled. Or, the lean meat and the egg may be cooked as an omelet.

Vegetables such as spinach, kale, broccoli, cauliflower, lettuce, green bean, cabbage, carrots, green pepper or corn may be boiled, steamed or stir-fried alone or with some lean meat, condiment, and vegetable oil.

Canned or dried apple, peach, grapefruit, orange, pear, and grapes are recommended instead of fresh fruit. Bananas are also a good choice due to their relatively low water content.

Hot water, tea, and coffee are recommended for drinks, but other beverages such as warm milk, almond milk, soy milk, and broth may be used. Sugar and honey may be added. A maximum of 6 ounces is recommended for the average person doing sedentary work.

The water factor (H_2O factor) may be estimated using the water content data from Table 1, Table 2, and Table 3. The water content for breakfast should be less than 75%.

Table 13. Lunch

Group	Food	Wt (oz)	H_2O factor	H_2O wt (oz)
Grain	Bread	4.00	0.37	1.48
	(or steamed rice)			
Meat	Grilled chicken	6.00	0.54	3.24
	(or fish, beef)			
Vegetable	Stir-fried cabbage	4.00	0.75	3.00
	Potato salad	3.00	0.68	2.04
Fruit	Canned	3.00	0.80	2.40
	(or preserved)			
Drinks	Hot water	8.00	1.00	8.00
	(or tea, coffee)			
Total	oz	28.00		20.16
	lbs	1.75		1.26
Water content				72%

Lunch may include selections from a variety of food groups. In the meat category, one may choose grilled chicken, pork, beef, turkey or fish. BBQ or baked chicken, pork, spare ribs, sausage, and steak would be good choices as well.

Any kind of vegetable may be boiled, steamed or stir-fried with some lean meat, condiment, and vegetable oil.

A hamburger, sandwich or hot dog with french fries or chips would be a good choice also.

Canned or dried fruits may be included in your lunch. Bananas are a healthy choice also.

Hot water, tea, and coffee may be selected for drinks. A maximum of 8 ounces is recommended for the average person doing sedentary work.

The water factor (H_2O factor) may be estimated using the water content data from Table 1, Table 2, and Table3. The water content for lunch should be less than 75%.

Table 14. Dinner

Group	Food	Wt (oz)	H_2O factor	H_2O wt (oz)
Grain	Steamed rice	4.00	0.63	2.52
	Bread	4.00	0.37	1.48
Meat	Roast beef	8.00	0.54	4.32
	(or fish, pork, chicken)			
Vegetable	Stir-fried broccoli	4.00	0.75	3.00
Fruit	Canned	4.00	0.80	3.20
	(or preserved)			
Drinks	Hot water	10.00	1.00	10.00
	(or tea, coffee)			
Total	oz	34.00		24.52
	lbs	2.13		1.53
Water content				72%

For dinner, any kind of lean meat would be acceptable. One may choose grilled chicken, pork, beef, turkey or fish. BBQ or baked chicken, pork, spare ribs, sausage, and steak would be good choices as well.

A variety of vegetables may be boiled, steamed or stir-fried with some lean meat, condiment, and vegetable oil. Baked or mashed potato with cheese and cream may be a good choice also.

Canned or dried fruits of any kind are recommended. Bananas may be selected as well.

Hot water, tea, and coffee may be chosen for drinks. Sugar, honey or milk is optional. A maximum of 10 oz. is recommended for the average person doing sedentary work.

The water factor (H_2O factor) may be estimated using the water content data from Table 1, Table 2, and Table 3. The water content for dinner should be less than 75%.

Table 15. Snacks

Group	Food	Wt (oz)	H_2O factor	H_2O wt (oz)
Grain	Cookies	4.00	0.07	0.14
Meat				
Vegetable				
Fruit	Dried	3.00	0.20	0.60
	(or canned)			
Drinks	Hot water	14.00	1.00	16.00
	(or tea, coffee)			
Total	oz	21.00		16.74
	lbs	1.31		1.05
Water content				80%

Snacks may include foods that are forbidden in most other diets. In the grain category, you may choose a cookie, cracker, donut, biscuit, chips, or cake due to their low water content. Small quantities of carbs are acceptable in this diet.

Instead of fresh fruits, choose canned or dried varieties. Bananas are the only exception.

One cup of hot tea or coffee in the morning and one in the afternoon should be sufficient for the snack.

18. Blank Diet Sheets

You can design meal plans using the following blank sheets.

Group	Food	Wt (oz)	H_2O factor	H_2O wt (oz)
Grain				
Meat				
Vegetable				
Fruit				
Drinks				
Total	oz			
	lbs			
Water content				%

Group	Food	Wt (oz)	H_2O factor	H_2O wt (oz)
Grain				
Meat				
Vegetable				
Fruit				
Drinks				
Total	oz			
	lbs			
Water content				%

Group	Food	Wt (oz)	H_2O factor	H_2O wt (oz)
Grain				
Meat				
Vegetable				
Fruit				
Drinks				
Total	oz			
	lbs			
Water content				%

Group	Food	Wt (oz)	H_2O factor	H_2O wt (oz)
Grain				
Meat				
Vegetable				
Fruit				
Drinks				
Total	oz			
	lbs			
Water content				%

Appendix E. Unit Conversion

Weight:

1	Pound	=	16	ounces (oz)
		=	453.6	grams (g)
		=	0.4536	kilograms (kg)
1	ounce	=	28.35	grams
1	kilogram	=	1,000	grams
		=	2.2	pounds (lbs)
		=	35.3	ounces
1	gram	=	0.0353	ounces

Volume:

1	US gallon	=	4	quarts
		=	8	pints
		=	3.785	liters (l)
		=	3,785	milliliters (cc)
		=	0.134	cubic feet
1	cubic feet	=	28.317	liters

Water Volume/Weight:

1	milliliter	=	1	gram
1	liter	=	1	kilogram
		=	1,000	grams
		=	0.264	gallons
1	US cup	=	8	ounces
1	glass	=	8	ounces
1	gallon	=	8.35	pounds

(6-pack 12 oz. can = 4.5 pounds)

Food Combustion Energy:

1	food calorie	=	1, 000	calories

Dr. Ching H. Wu

Dr. Wu was born and raised in Miaoli, Taiwan. His education and training were completed in Taiwan and in the United States. Dr. Wu has earned degrees in engineering and Traditional Chinese Medicine. Over the years, he worked as a mining engineer, geologist, petroleum engineer, chemical engineer, college professor, acupuncturist, and Chinese herbalist.

In the early 1990's, Dr. Wu's interest in life evolved from teaching engineering to alleviating human suffering. He has helped many patients with obesity, fibromyalgia, cancer, asthma, chronic and seasonal allergies, rheumatism, migraines, bipolar disorder, skin disorders, depression, sport injuries, and auto injuries.

Dr. Wu wrote the Low-Water High-Energy Weight Loss Plan in hopes of helping many to maintain optimum weight and good health.

- Diploma Mining Engineering, Taipei Institute of Technology
- MS Petroleum Engineering, Colorado School of Mines
- PhD Chemical and Petroleum Engineering, University of Pittsburgh
- Senior Chemical Engineer, Texaco Bellaire Laboratory
- Associate Professor, Colorado School of Mines
- Professor, Texas A&M University
- Diploma Oriental Medicine, Texas Institute of Oriental Medicine
- MS TCM, Texas College of Traditional Chinese Medicine
- Diplomate in Acupuncture, NCCAOM
- Proprietor, Wu's Acupuncture and Herbs
- Licensed acupuncturist. Oregon (AC00667); Texas (Ex - AC00038)

9 780615 841731